YOUR KNOWLEDGE HAS VALUE

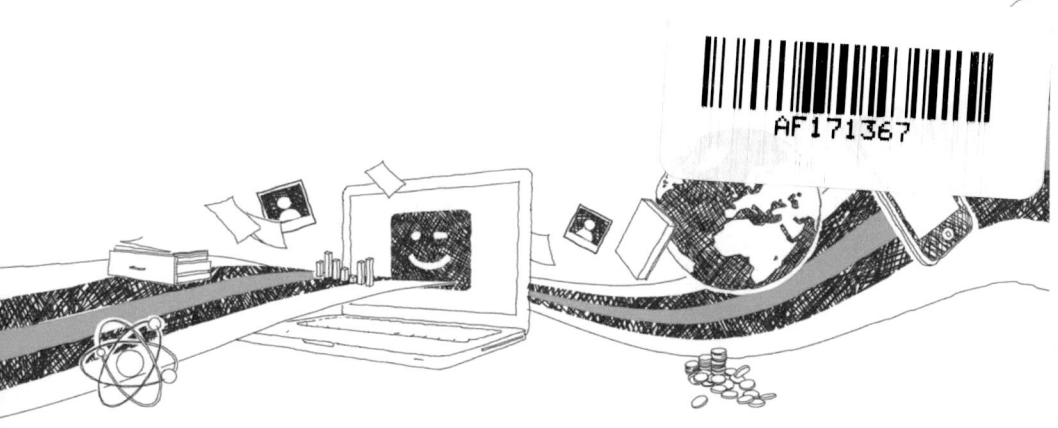

- We will publish your bachelor's and master's thesis, essays and papers

- Your own eBook and book - sold worldwide in all relevant shops

- Earn money with each sale

Upload your text at www.GRIN.com
and publish for free

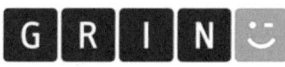

Bibliographic information published by the German National Library:

The German National Library lists this publication in the National Bibliography; detailed bibliographic data are available on the Internet at http://dnb.dnb.de .

This book is copyright material and must not be copied, reproduced, transferred, distributed, leased, licensed or publicly performed or used in any way except as specifically permitted in writing by the publishers, as allowed under the terms and conditions under which it was purchased or as strictly permitted by applicable copyright law. Any unauthorized distribution or use of this text may be a direct infringement of the author s and publisher s rights and those responsible may be liable in law accordingly.

Imprint:

Copyright © 2018 GRIN Verlag
Print and binding: Books on Demand GmbH, Norderstedt Germany
ISBN: 9783346034663

This book at GRIN:

https://www.grin.com/document/501988

Erick Otieno, Freida Mutui, Michael Okuku

Risk Management on Water and Sanitation

GRIN Verlag

GRIN - Your knowledge has value

Since its foundation in 1998, GRIN has specialized in publishing academic texts by students, college teachers and other academics as e-book and printed book. The website www.grin.com is an ideal platform for presenting term papers, final papers, scientific essays, dissertations and specialist books.

Visit us on the internet:

http://www.grin.com/

http://www.facebook.com/grincom

http://www.twitter.com/grin_com

Risk Management Strategies and Performance of Kosovo Water and Sanitation Project, Nairobi County Kenya.
Erick Otieno

Content

ABSTRACT 1
STUDY BACKGROUND 1
RESEARCH METHODOLOGY 5
RESULTS AND DISCUSSIONS 5
CONCLUSSION AND RECOMMENDATION 9
REFERENCES 10

ABSTRACT
The purpose of this study was to present the systematic risk evaluation based of literature on the practice of risk management strategies on water and sanitation and how this affects the lives of Kosovo village informal settlement. The risk which comes along with these projects are mainly fatal waterborne infectious diseases which results to death. This challenge occurs mainly when the project lacks comprehensive risk evaluation plan and the methods employed in risk mitigation are not efficient to control such adverse effects. The purpose of this research was to determine the relationship between the risk avoidance strategy and the performance of Kosovo water and sanitation project in Nairobi county. A mixed method research was involved in the study which elaborate data collection and data analysis. Both quantitative and qualitative data was integrated in a single study. A mixed method research approach and descriptive survey design was employed in the study. The sample size was determined using Kjercie & Morgan (1970) sample size determination table. The sample size coinciding to the population of 260 was 152. Purposive sampling was used to select the 155 members of the households from the population. Questionnaires comprised of closed and open-ended questions were administered so that to allow the population to express their opinion based on the experience on water and sanitation related diseases infection risks. The quantitative data analysis was carried out using descriptive statistics by use of Statistical Package for Social Science (SPSS). The descriptive statistics entailed use of measure of central tendency and percentages. Presentation of the results was carried out using tables, charts and figures. The study found out that there has been little effort made by the county government and stakeholders to mitigate the risk effects. There are no adequate toilets in the area and human waste are disposed in ways that are prone to spread diseases. The bathrooms are paid for and at least ten households share one bathroom. Sewer pipes are located in the same place with the water pipes, in case the water pipe develops leakage or bursts, the waste is absorbed in the water pipes and this transports infections to the tap water used in the households. Waste are disposed in the nearby Nairobi river which becomes flooded with paper bags. This also results to spread of mosquito which bring along malaria infections. It is thus recommended that the county government of Nairobi should initiative building toilets and construct sewages in Kosovo. This will take place first by involving the community through effective training on skills to mitigate risks. Policies of sanitation and waste disposal should be formulated in line with the water and sanitation policies which guides the community on risk management practices.

Key words: Project, Risk, Risk management, Risk avoidance, community Involvement.

STUDY BACKGROUND
Risk in a project is measured on likelihood and consequences that arises during the projects course Project cost and time overran occurs due to lack of measurement system for assessing and controlling project risks. Risk events are controlled in a sequence of steps whose objectives are to perceive, address, and remove chance objects earlier than they become either threats to a success operation (Oltadel, Moen & Clempe, 2004). The aim of this research was to understand how the risk avoidance strategy relates to the performance of Kosovo water and sanitation project in Nairobi county. Access to safe drinking water and sanitation is a global concern, especially as a millennium development goal. This has been mainly addressed as one of the basic

global human rights. Over billion people around the globe do not have sufficient access to clean water and sanitation (He & Charlet, 2013). The escalating water and sanitation risk disaster constitutes a threat for worldwide progress towards sustainable improvement in the new millennium. The Global Burden of Disease Study undertaken by the World Bank indicates that 15% water borne diseases in children under 5 years in African countries are directly attributable to diarrheal disease. Eighty-eight percent of these disease burden is caused by the risk of unsafe sanitation, water, and hygiene (Philippines & Luzon). The deepening risk disaster in water and sanitation worldwide is particularly acute problem in countries and remains a primary challenge. In many urban slums, safe consuming water from an advanced supply and sanitation offerings remain unacceptably insufficient (WHO-UNICEF,2014). In 2001, more than one million children in Sub-Saharan Africa died of conditions related to unsafe water and sanitation (APHRC, 2012). Availability of clean water and sanitation projects owing to their complex nature are beset with risks which if not systematically managed causes projects to result into many negative impacts than the expected benefits. Occurrence of the risk of water-borne diseases and diarrhea have been largely attributed to by inadequate vis-à-vis water quality in the Ibadan city on Nigeria where 1,334 cases were collected from eight public hospitals. Water samples were also collected from different sources in order to refer to for the water and sanitation disease related cases. The application of domestic water treatment methods such as bottling become one of the best ways to avoid the intending risks of water borne diseases. According to the European Center for Disease and Control, the most immediate risk face by the European Union travelers in the affected areas of Zimbabwe, Malawi and Mozambique are related to the direct transmission of diarrheal diseases due to the risk of lack of drinking or contaminated water and poor sanitation in the region. The overall risk of water and sanitation in this area lowered when the European group offered to launch few water projects and sanitation improvements in the area (Williams,2017) This informs the critical management of the potential risks by identifying, analyzing and addressing them to reduce the probability or impact of unfavorable negative events and maximize realization of emerging opportunities.

Risk management outcome may help to mitigate the likelihood of risk occurring and the negative impact when occurs. For instance, risk management can be a barrier to eradication of poverty. In Uganda, 50% do not have access to clean water, while 40% do not have sanitation facilities. The need of water is significant and due to the distance to the sources, people get attempt to use the nearby contaminated water sources which results to dangerous diseases in Bukiwe district in Uganda (WHO,2015).

The Kenyan vision 2030 points out that, Kenya has scarcity of water with renewable sparkling water in step with capita at 647 m3 towards the united nations encouraged minimal of one,1000 m3. For the reason that water is a scarce resource, it raises the query of challenge design, making plans and implementation strategies of water initiatives that may improve the livelihoods of the people. It is consequently vital to decide the results of water and sanitation venture variables at the livelihoods of slum dwellers which include their socio financial and cultural welfare in addition to the environmental situation of their habitats with minimal risk impacts. Kenya loses 25 billion shillings every year due to annually due to poor sanitation (Water & Sanitation Program report; March 2012). According to the Millennium Project's Task Force on Water and Sanitation, sufficient water access is the ability to obtain sufficient quantities of water that are safe to drink and available for hygienic purposes (Abrar, 2018). Some of the Kosovo water sources where health risks evolve include: piped water into dwelling, public tap or standpipe with the inconsistent quality with frequent contamination from vandalized pipes and shut-offs. (Mshida, 2017).

Risk management has become an important part of the management process for any project. (Akintoye & MacLeod, 2013), believes that health crisis within the society had led to adopting risk management and analysis into practice. Project risk management has a prominent position in the framework of project management theory and methodology. The reason is that unexpected events will usually occur during a project. Given the importance of project risk management in project management functioning, the efficiency of risk management is expected to significantly influence project performance.

Statement of the problem
Access to safe drinking water and adequate sanitation in urban areas is likely to worsen unless there is a drastic policy change for risk mitigation strategies in order to cater for the needs of the urban poor. In Kenya there have been various water and sanitation project initiatives from Nairobi county government and development agencies to improve the living conditions of individuals dwelling in the informal settlements. These include mostly a range of clean water provision and safe sanitation. Although the Kosovo village has experienced a single implementation of water and sanitation project, little is known about the risk implications to the livelihood of Kosovo residents. The risks brought by water results into cholera epidemics, faecal-oral illnesses like symptom, and occurrence of malaria which results to the rise of disease and mortality rates. This means that risk impact evaluation has never been done effectively for whatever reason. Despite the improvement of the informal settlement livelihood in Kosovo slum, the county government and development agencies have been reluctant to carry out evaluation because they deemed to be technically complex and findings can be politically sensitive especially if the results are negative. There exists no study that has ever focused on documenting such risks brought along by water and sanitation projects in Kosovo slum. The study was done particularly to determine and critically evaluate the effectiveness of risk avoidance strategy on the performance of Kosovo water and sanitation project as the modest attempt to bridge this gap.

Risk Avoidance Strategy on Water and Sanitation Project
When a risk is identified during the project implementation, it sets an intention on the project to be set on the exposure to the uncertain situations. A project can be associated with various opportunities and threats at the same time. For instance water and sanitation project will bring water availability and a health relief to the community which will be perceived as a positive impact, however the uncertainties encountered and the pending risks will be counted as threats to the community and dangerous to human health (Phillipines, Luzon, 2011).

Avoiding the project in case the risk negative impacts outweighs the project opportunities will lead to more risk of diseases. According to the WHO (2014), the provision of good water and sanitation to the community leads to poverty alleviation and improve productivity. Community can decide on corporate social responsibility that help to build the social dimension by demonstrating corporate action in order to meet social and environmental expectations of the stakeholders to maintain future social corporation. This also increase public participation in the community-based project and supports the decision making on what suits the community. If the danger is assessed as a transportation to negative consequences to the total project, it's of importance to review the project's aim (Oltedal, Moen, Klempe, & Rundmo, 2004). In different words, if the danger has vital impact on the project, the most effective resolution is to avoid it by dynamical the scope of the project or, worst state of affairs or cancel it. There are several potential risks that water and sanitation projects become exposed to, and which may impact its success (Lee, Workman & Jung, 2016). This brings out a necessary action and why risk management is significant within the early stages of a project rather than coping with the harm when the incidence of the danger.

By having an overview over the whole project, it is easy to identify problems which are causing damage to the water and sanitation project.

In Roll back malaria project across Africa, established in 1998, the project did not meet it objectives because donors at no extent followed their pledges of the amount of money required per year. The infection rate went higher, and the project resulted to be not of beneficial. The experts may find solutions that the project team has not considered (Katulanga, Amaratunga, & Parvez, 2010). Risk avoidance means that by looking at alternatives in the project, a risk can be eliminated. If major changes are required in the project in order to avoid risks application of known and well-developed strategies instead of new ones, even if the new ones may appear to be more cost efficient. In this way, the risks can be avoided, and work can proceed smoothly because strategy is less stressful to the users. For instance, the failure of Chad-Cameroon oil pipeline to the Atlantic Ocean in 2003 resulted due to lack of economic risk avoidance and the projects funds were diverted to a different channel of government development (Williams,2017). Risk avoidance involves changing the project plan to eliminate the risk or the condition that causes the risk in order to protect the project objectives from its impact. This may be either by eliminating the source of risk within a project or by avoiding projects. Eliminating activities with a high probability of loss by making it difficult for risk to occur, or by executing the project in a different way which will achieve the same objectives, but which insulates the project from the effect of the risk can be termed was risk avoidance. Some activities that can help to avoid potential risk: more detailed planning, alternative approaches, protection and safety systems, operation reviews, regular inspections, training and skills enhancement, permits to work and procedural changes. Preventive maintenance.

Communication between project head and management is crucial to the successful implementation of project. This is generally influenced by the principal agent relationship between the parties and the contract type. shows that a balance between formal and informal communication between project manager and other stakeholders reduces mistrust and conflict of interest. The importance of project managers' skills and leadership capabilities, user involvement, top management commitment and organizational engagement leads to successful implementation of projects. Weak links between project stakeholders affect the effectiveness of project governance state that among many reasons behind project failure, planning fallacy, i.e., over-optimism in the planning phase in the project due to resource misallocation and miscommunication is crucial. It is preferable if a project is budgeted, one phase at a time, instead of budgeting all at once time. (Al-ansari & Adamo, 2018).

Initiating community activities like dissemination of disaster risk data, conveyancing early warnings to their peers, and involvement of the authorities are allotted by Community Based Social Organizations. This means that these CBSOs, through their social networks, will become active agents of amendment and bridge the communication gap between government and community. Thus, CBSOs' risk communication provides the chance to contribute to the general resilience-building and disaster risk avoidance as a part of people-centered actions and native responses to risk disaster (Hilson, 2014).

Periodic communication of risk assessment results can mitigate risks in projects. Risk assessments are repositories of structured information and a medium for communication. Hence, the judicious use of risk assessment tools with adequate communication can mitigate risks to a great extent (Abrar, 2018). Internal communication is one of the most important factors for success in project management. Project manager should tract the internal communication to ensure project deliverables to make ends meet. Avoiding risk can sometimes be a limitation to the likelihood of other possible opportunities.

RESEARCH METHODOLOGY

A mixed method research approach was adopted in this study. The target population in this study was 260households in Kosovo village Nairobi county. A descriptive survey research design was adopted in this study. The sample size for the study was determine by use of Krejcie & Morgan (1970) sample size table. The sample size corresponding to 300 was 152 households. Purposive sampling was used to select 152 adult members from the target population. A total of 117(76.2%) of the anticipated respondents participated in the study. Data collection was carried out using questionnaires. The quantitative data was analyzed using SPSS software to obtain results. Qualitative data was analyzed using thematic analysis and presentation of the results in prose form. Findings are presented by use of charts, figures and tables. The correlation analysis explained the relationship between risk avoidance strategy and the performance of Kosovo water and sanitation project.

RESULTS AND DISCUSSIONS

Descriptive statistics for Risk Avoidance Strategy and performance of water and sanitation project.

This objective sought to determine the relationship between risk avoidance strategy and the performance of Kosovo water and sanitation project in Nairobi county. The statements were presented in a scale of 1-5, **where 1- Highly Disagree, 2- Disagree, 3- Neutral, 4- Agree, 5- Highly Agree.**

Table 4.1 Risk avoidance strategy

	Highly Disagree (%)	Disagree (%)	Neutral (%)	Agree (%)	Highly Agree (%)	Mean	Std. Deviation
Community involvement to avoid future water borne disease risks.	12	18.8	6	26.5	38.5	3.64	1.417
Both men and women are involved in the risk avoidance process against water related illness.	7	9.4	17.1	25.6	41.9	3.88	1.226
Risk avoidance involves every household in setting the measures.	22	6	10.3	23.1	41.9	3.63	1.529
Risk avoidance will protect family members from water and sanitation related disease risks.	5	6.8	10.3	18.8	59.8	4.23	1.148

The above table shows that community involvement is a major initiative to avoid water borne disease related risks. The study findings indicated that 10.3% (12) highly disagreed to the statement of involving community. This is due to the insignificant number of Kosovo village members who rarely participate in the community building. 18.8% (22) disagreed because this also contains a number of individuals including women who believes that only certain group in the community is able to participate in risk management, while 6.0% (7) remained neutral about the situation. This showed that most of the Kosovo members are not aware of the intending risks and considers some innless brought about by this risk as normal. 26.5% (31) agreed and the 38.5% constituted of (45) respondents highly agreed. This indicated that majority of residents of Kosovo village highly supports involving community in the water project will be a great initiative that will resolve the risk situation brought along by water and sanitation project in

Kosovo slum. Findings from the analyzed data concerning both gender involvement indicates that (41.9%) of the respondents highly agreed with the statement that community involvement in water and sanitation project will be a better way to avoid water and sanitation disease risks. (25.6%) of the respondents agreed, 17.1% were neutral and 9.4% disagreed. The analysis from involving both men and women in project risk avoidance indicates that 25.6% which constitutes 30 agreed that both gender participation. 41.9% which constitutes 49 highly agreed with men and women participation as a risk management strategy. 17.1 % remains neutral, that is 20 members of Kosovo slum residents while 6.0% that constitutes 7 highly disagreed. The community is highly at agreement that women and men should apply equal effort towards achieving the risk avoidance strategies.

The analysis on the statement regarding households reveals that 23.1% which constitutes 27 agreed that involving every household in risk management will be a suitable way for cubing the risk. 41.9% which constitutes 49 highly agreed while 10.3% which constitutes 12 remains neutral. 18.8% highly disagreed which constitutes 22 and the remaining 6.0% disagreed that involving every household in risk management will be a better way to avoid the events of risks in water and sanitation project. The data analysis also concerning family members health in relation to the risk situation observes that 59.8% which constitutes 70 households highly agreed that risk avoidance will be a suitable way to protect all the families in every households against the infectious disease. 18.8% which constitutes of 22 agrees that this process will protect all families against water borne related diseases. 10.3% which constitutes of 12 remained neutral while 6.8% disagreed. 4.3% that constitutes of 5 highly disagreed that risk avoidance will protect every family from water related diseases. Avoiding the water and sanitation disease related risks such as cholera and typhoid will also enhance the productivity of the water users. This will enhance the participation of community members while initiating other uses of water for economic income such as opening car wash business and also ability to sell clean water for drinking for economic improvement.

Correlation Between Risk Avoidance Strategy and Project Performance

Table 4.5 Correlation between risk avoidance strategies and performance of Kosovo water and sanitation project.

		Community involvement in Kosovo water and sanitation project is a major initiative to avoid water borne disease risks	Project identified both men and women should be involved in the risk avoidance process against water related diseases risks	Risk avoidance is a process that should involve every household in setting the measures to control water related disease health risks	Risk avoidance will protect family members against the suffering from water and sanitation related disease risks
Community involvement to avoid water borne disease risks.	Pearson Correlation	1	0.094	.265**	0.099
	Sig. (2-tailed)		0.313	0.004	0.288
	N	117	117	117	117
Both men and women should be involved in the risk avoidance process.	Pearson Correlation	0.094	1	0.105	.240**
	Sig. (2-tailed)	0.313		0.259	0.009
	N	117	117	117	117
Risk avoidance is a process that should involve every household in setting the measures to control water and sanitation risks	Pearson Correlation	.265**	0.105	1	0.014
	Sig. (2-tailed)	0.004	0.259		0.878
	N	117	117	117	117
Risk avoidance will protect family members against water and sanitation related disease risks.	Pearson Correlation	0.099	.240**	0.014	1
	Sig. (2-tailed)	0.288	0.009	0.878	
	N	117	117	117	117

** Correlation is significant at the 0.01 level (2-tailed).

According to the table 4.5, the presented data serves as indication to what type and strength and relationships between the risk avoidance strategy and the performance of Kosovo water and sanitation project in Nairobi county using two-tailed tests. The analysis indicated a positive strong relationship (r) 0.094 and value of (p)0.313 between risk avoidance strategy and the performance of Kosovo water and sanitation project. The implication is that the application of risk avoidance strategies increases to an equal proportion with the performance. This means that the application of risk avoidance strategy will improve the performance of the water and sanitation project. There was a weak positive correlation of (r) 0.313 and (p) 0.094 between involving men and women in risk avoidance process and the performance of Kosovo water and sanitation project. This showed that either of the gender participation will have significant in the project. The situation here assumes that men participation in this activity can be much of significance as well as if both genders are combined. Men countered this idea that women mostly play little role in the decision making when it comes to planning for risk avoidance in this livelihood setting.

These was significantly strong positive correlation of (r) 0.004 and (p) 265 between the statement that risk avoidance should involve every household setting in order to come up with a critical solution to avoid the intending risks in water and sanitation usage. The use of water and sanitation is this settlement is estimated by the number of households so the number of households will determine the usage of water capacity. There is a weak positive correlation of (r) 0.099 and (p) 0.288 between the statement of risk avoidance will protect the family members against suffering from water and sanitation related disease infections. This relationship shows that many of the families disagreed with this statement because there have been risks in the water and sanitation project which people survive with. This are such as consuming unclean water and us of cure such as medical prescriptions for treatment.

Summary of Findings
The objective sought to assess the relationship between risk avoidance strategy and the performance of Kosovo water and sanitation project in Nairobi county. The mean obtained from the result was 3.64 and standard deviation of 1.417. The project involvement of community in water and sanitation is a great initiative and this will to a greater extent enable risk avoidance to become effective and manageable. Recognizing men and women in the risk management has been agreed at 41.9% meaning that both members of the society has a role in the project initiative. Information concerning risks to the households being made aware is significant because this enables people learn ways to take caution against contaminated waters and waster disposal. This has been highly agreed at 41.9% meaning that the household members support the initiation in risk avoidance process. 59.8% has also agreed that if the water and sanitation related risks are avoided, this will save lives and to the better results of risk mitigation practices.

CONCLUSSION AND RECOMMENDATION

This study sought to determine the relationship between the risk avoidance strategy and the performance of Kosovo water and sanitation project in Nairobi county. From the findings, the study revealed that community involvement, equal gender participation and set policies on water use have direct influence on risk avoidance in the project. On this basis, the study recommends that the county government and ministry of water should back up on the risk mitigation concerning water and sanitation utilization will be ideal initiatives to avoid water and sanitation intended disease risks.

REFERENCES

Abrar, H., Hussain, S. J., Chaudhry, J., Saleem, K., Orgun, M. A., Al-, J., & Valli, C. (2018). Risk Analysis of Cloud Sourcing in Healthcare and Public Health Industry. *IEEE Acess*, 6(February), 11. https://doi.org/10.1109/ACCESS.2018.2805919.

Akintoye, A. S., & MacLeod, M. J. (2003). Risk analysis and management in construction. International Journal of Project Management, 15(1), 31–38. https://doi.org/10.1016/S0263-7863(96)00035-X.

Al-ansari, N., & Adamo, N. (2018). Present Water Crises in Iraq and Its Human and Environmental Implications. Scientific Research Publishing Inc, 10(4), 305–319. https://doi.org/10.4236/eng.2018.106021.

Bhoola, V., Hiremath, S. B., & MAllik, D. (2014). An Assessment of Risk Response Strategies Practiced in Software Projects. Australasian Journal of Information Systems, 18(3), 161–191.

Cutter, S. L., Lavell, A., Burton, I., & Oliver-Smith, A. (2014). Governance in Disaster Risk Management (IRDR.

He, J., & Charlet, L. (2013). A review of Arsenic Presence in China Drinking Water. JournalofHydrology,492(10),79–88. https://doi.org/10.1016/j.jhydrol.2013.04.007

Hillson, D. (2014). Using a Risk Breakdown Structure in Project Management. Facilities Management, 2(1), 85–97. https://doi.org/10.1108/14725960410808131.

Kulatunga, U., Amaratunga, D., Science, P., Parvez, A., & Science, P. (2010). Community risk assessment for disaster risk reduction : challenges and future.

Lee, S., Workman, J. E., & Jung, K. (2016). Brand Relationships and Risk : Influence of risk Avoidance and Gender on Brand Consumption. Open Innovation: Technology, Market, and Complexity, 14(2), 15. https://doi.org/10.1186/s40852-016-0041-0

Mshida, H. A., Kassim, N., Kimanya, M. E., & Mpolya, E. (2017). Influence of Water , Sanitation , and Hygiene Practices on Common Infections among Under-Five Children in Longido and Monduli Districts of Arusha , Tanzania. Journal of Environmental and Public Health, 2017(ID 9235168), 8.

Oltedal, S., Moen, B., Klempe, H., & Rundmo, T. (2004). Explaining Risk Perception An Evaluation of Cultural Theory.

Phillipines, Luzon, C. (2011). Disaster Risk Management for Health, Saniattion and Hygiene. United Kingdom.

WHO-UNICEF. (2014). Joint Monitoring Program for Water and Sanitation.

http://www.wssinfo.org/en/238_wat_latino.html

Williams, T. (2017). The Nature of Risk in Complex Projects. Project Management Journal, 48(4), 55–66.

Whittaker, A., & Taylor, B. (2017). Understanding Risk in Social Work. *Journal of Social Work Practice*, *31*(4), 375–378. https://doi.org/10.1080/02650533.2017.1397612

YOUR KNOWLEDGE HAS VALUE

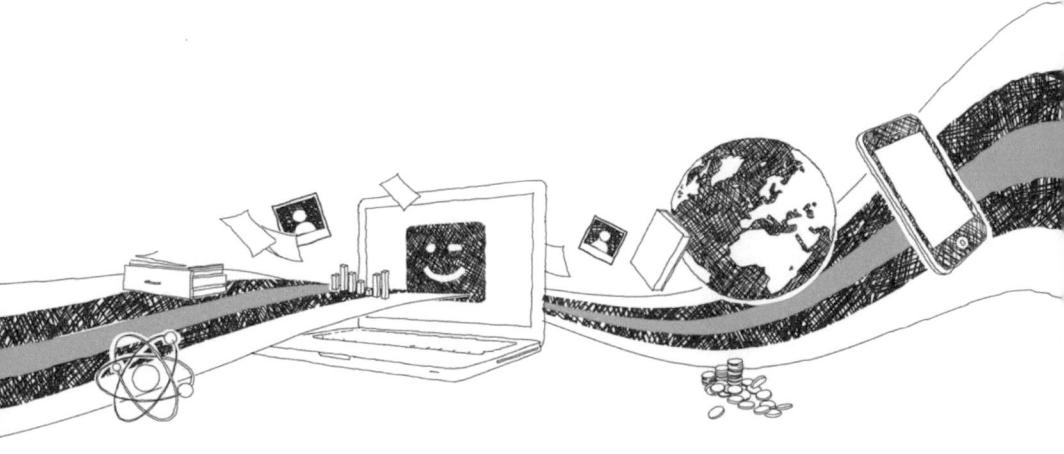

- We will publish your bachelor's and master's thesis, essays and papers

- Your own eBook and book - sold worldwide in all relevant shops

- Earn money with each sale

Upload your text at www.GRIN.com
and publish for free

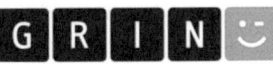